The Plant-Based Way to Dinner

The Best Collection of Dinner Recipes to Start Your Plant-Based Diet and Improve Your Lifestyle

W0010116

Dave Ingram

© Copyright 2020 - All rights reserved.

The content contained within this book may not be reproduced, duplicated or transmitted without direct written permission from the author or the publisher.

Under no circumstances will any blame or legal responsibility be held against the publisher, or author, for any damages, reparation, or monetary loss due to the information contained within this book. Either directly or indirectly.

Legal Notice:

This book is copyright protected. This book is only for personal use. You cannot amend, distribute, sell, use, quote or paraphrase any part, or the content within this book, without the consent of the author or publisher.

Disclaimer Notice:

Please note the information contained within this document is for educational and entertainment purposes only. All effort has been executed to present accurate, up to date, and reliable, complete information. No warranties of any kind are declared or implied. Readers acknowledge that the author is not engaging in the rendering of legal, financial, medical or professional advice. The content within this book has been derived from various sources. Please consult a licensed professional before attempting any techniques outlined in this book.

By reading this document, the reader agrees that under no circumstances is the author responsible for any losses, direct or indirect, which are incurred as a result of the use of information contained within this document, including, but not limited to, — errors, omissions, or inaccuracies.

Table of contents

3

Barbecued Greens & Grits

Preparation Time: 20 minutes

Cooking Time: 4 hours

Servings: 4

Ingredients:

14 oz. tempeh, sliced 3 cups vegetable broth

3 cups collard greens, chopped

½ cup BBQ sauce

1   cup gluten-free grits

¼ cup white onion, diced

2   tbsps. olive oil

2 garlic cloves, minced 1 tsp. salt

Directions:

1.   Preheat the oven to 400°F.

2.   Mix tempeh slices with the BBQ sauce in a shallow baking dish. Set aside and let marinate for up to 3 hours.

3.   Heat 1 tsp of olive oil in a frying pan over medium heat and then add the garlic and sauté until it is fragrant.

4.   Add the collard greens and ½ teaspoon of salt and cook until the collards are wilted and dark. Set the pan from heat and set it aside.

5.   Cover the tempeh and BBQ sauce mixture with aluminum foil. In your oven, set the baking dish in place and bake the ingredients for 15 minutes. Uncover and continue to bake for another 10 minutes until the tempeh is browned and crispy.

6.   While the tempeh cooks, heat the remaining tablespoon of olive oil in the previously used frying pan over medium heat.

7.   Cook the onions until brown and fragrant, around 10 minutes.

8.   Pour in the vegetable broth, bring it to a boil, then turn the heat down to low.

9.   Slowly whisk the grits into the simmering broth. Add the remaining ½ teaspoon of salt before covering the pan with a lid.

10.   Let the ingredients simmer for about 8 minutes until the grits are soft and creamy.

11.   Serve the tempeh and collard greens on top of a bowl of grits and enjoy, or store for later!

Nutrition: Calories: 374, Fat: 19.1g, Carbs: 31.1g, Protein: 23.7g

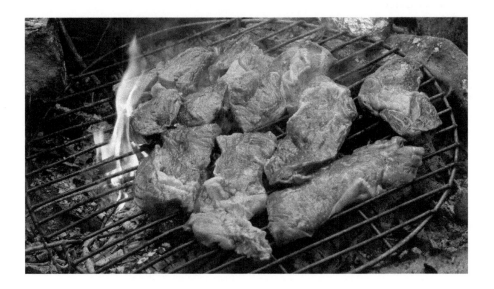

Chickpea and Spinach Cutlets

Preparation Time: 10 minutes

Cooking Time: 30 minutes

Servings: 12

Ingredients:

1 Red Bell Pepper

19 oz. Chickpeas, Rinsed & Drained 1 cup ground Almonds

2 tsps. Dijon Mustard 1 tsp. Oregano

½ tsp. Sage

1 cup Spinach, Fresh 1½ cup Rolled Oats

1   Clove Garlic, Pressed

½ Lemon, Juiced

2   tsps. Maple Syrup, Pure

Directions:

1.   Get out a baking sheet. Line it with parchment paper.

2.   Cut your red pepper in half, and then take the seeds out. Place it on your baking sheet and roast it in the oven while you prepare your other ingredients.

3.   Process your chickpeas, almonds, mustard, and maple syrup together in a food processor.

4.   Add in your lemon juice, oregano, sage, garlic, and spinach, processing again. Make sure it's combined, but don't puree it.

5.   Once your red bell pepper is softened, which should roughly take ten minutes, add this to the processor as well. Add in your oats, mixing well.

6.   Form twelve patties, cooking in the oven for a half-hour. They should be browned.

Nutrition: Calories: 200 Protein: 8g

Fat: 11g Carbs: 21g

Flavorful Refried Beans

Preparation Time: 10 minutes

Cooking Time: 6 hours

Servings: 8

Ingredients:

3   cups rinsed pinto beans

1   seeded jalapeno pepper, chopped 1 sliced white onion, peeled

2   tbsps. Minced garlic 5 tsps. salt

2 tsps. Ground black pepper

¼ tsps. ground cumin 9 cups water

Directions:

1.   Using a 6-quart slow cooker, place all the ingredients and stir until it mixes properly.

2.   Cover the top, plug in the slow cooker, adjust the cooking time to 6 hours, let it cook on a high heat setting, and add more water if the beans get too dry.

3.   When beans are done, drain and reserve the liquid.

4.   Mash the beans and pour in the reserved cooking liquid until it reaches your desired mixture.

Nutrition:

Calories: 105 Carbs: 36g Protein:13g Fat:1g

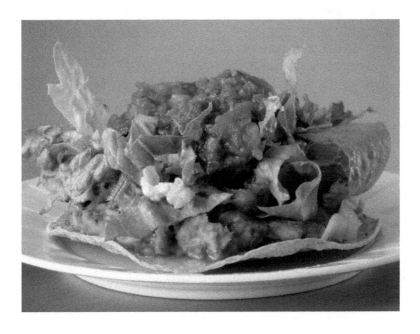

Smoky Red Beans and Rice

Preparation Time: 10 minutes

Cooking Time: 4 hours

Servings: 6

Ingredients:

30 oz. cooked red beans

1 cup rice

1 cup pepper

1 cup chopped celery

1 cup white onion, chopped 1 ½ tbsp. Minced garlic

½ tsp. salt

¼ tsp. Cayenne pepper 1 tsp. Smoked paprika 2 tsps. dried thyme

1   bay leaf

2   1/3 cups vegetable broth

Directions:

1.   Using a 6-quart slow cooker, place all the ingredients except for the rice, salt, and cayenne pepper.

2.   Stir until it mixes appropriately, and then cover the top.

3.   Plug in the slow cooker, adjust the cooking time to 4 hours, and steam on a low heat setting.

4.   Then pour in and stir the rice, salt, cayenne pepper and continue cooking for an additional 2 hours at a high heat setting.

Nutrition:

Calories: 425 Carbs: 62g Protein: 27g Fat: 22g

Savory Spanish Rice

Preparation Time: 5 minutes

Cooking Time: 5 hours

Servings: 10

Ingredients:

1 cup long-grain rice, uncooked

½ cup green bell pepper, chopped 14 oz. Diced tomatoes

½ cup chopped white onion 1 tsp. Minced garlic

½ tsp. salt

1 tsp. Red chili powder 1 tsp. ground cumin

4   oz. Tomato puree 8 fl. oz. water

Directions:

1.   Grease a 6-quart slow cooker with a non-stick cooking spray and add all the ingredients into it.

2.   Stir properly and cover the top.

3.   Plug in the slow cooker; adjust the cooking time to 5 hours, and cook on high or until the rice absorbs all the liquid.

Nutrition:

Calories: 210 Cal, Carbs: 11g, Protein: 12g, Fat: 10g

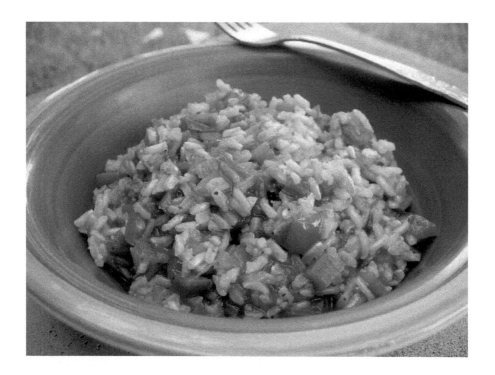

Delightful Coconut Vegetarian Curry

Preparation Time: 10 minutes

Cooking Time: 5 hours

Servings: 6

Ingredients:

5   potatoes, peeled and cubed

¼ cup curry powder 2 tbsps. flour

1 tbsp. Chili powder

½ tsp. Red pepper flakes

½ tsp. cayenne pepper

1 green pepper

1 red pepper

2   tbsps. onion soup mix

14 oz. coconut cream, unsweetened

3 cups vegetable broth

2 carrots

1 cup peas

¼ cup chopped cilantro

Directions:

1.   Take a 6-quart slow cooker, grease it with a non-stick cooking spray and place the potatoes pieces in the bottom.

2.   Set in the rest of the ingredients except for peas, cilantro, and carrots.

3.   Stir properly and cover the top.

4.   Plug in the slow cooker; adjust the cooking time to 4 hours and let it cook on the low heat setting or until it cooks thoroughly.

5.   When the cooking time is over, add the carrots to the curry and continue cooking for 30 minutes.

6.   Stir in the peas to cook for 30 more minutes or until the peas get tender.

7.   Garnish it with cilantro and serve.

Nutrition: Calories: 369 Carbs: 39g, Protein: 7g, Fat: 23g

Beauty School Ginger Cucumbers

Preparation Time: 10 minutes

Cooking Time: 45 minutes

Servings: 14

Ingredients:

1 sliced cucumber

3 tsp. Rice wine vinegar 1 ½ tbsp. sugar

1 tsp. minced ginger

Directions:

1.   Place all together with the ingredients in a mixing bowl, and toss the ingredients well. Enjoy!

Nutrition: Calories: 10 kcal Protein: 0.46 g Fat: 0.43 g Carbohydrates: 0.89 g

Exotic Butternut Squash and Chickpea Curry

Preparation Time: 20 minutes

Cooking Time: 6 hours

Servings: 8

Ingredients:

1 1/2 cups of shelled peas

1 1/2 cups of chickpeas, uncooked and rinsed 2 1/2 cups of diced butternut squash

12 ounce of chopped spinach 2 large tomatoes, diced

1 small white onion, peeled and chopped 1 teaspoon of minced garlic

1 teaspoon of salt

3 tablespoons of curry powder 14-ounce of coconut milk

3 cups of vegetable broth 1/4 cup of chopped cilantro

Directions:

1.   Using a 6-quart slow cooker, place all the ingredients into it except for the spinach and peas.

2.   Cover the top, plug in the slow cooker, adjust the cooking time to 6 hours, and cook on the high heat setting until the chickpeas get tender.

3.   30 minutes to ending your cooking, add the peas and spinach to the slow cooker and cook for the remaining 30 minutes.

4.   Stir to check the sauce; if the sauce is runny, stir in a mixture of 1 tbsp. Cornstarch mixed with 2 tbsp. Water.

5.   Serve with boiled rice.

Nutrition: Calories: 774 kcal Protein: 3.71 g Fat: 83.25 g Carbohydrates: 12.64 g

Kind-to-Cows Seitan

Servings: 6 (4 ounces, or 113 g each)

Ingredients:

For the seitan:

1 ¼ cups (180 g) vital wheat gluten 3 tablespoons (23 g) chickpea flour

1 tablespoon (10 g) granulated tapioca

1 tablespoon (7 g) onion powder 1 teaspoon garlic powder

½ teaspoon ground black pepper

¼ cup (180 ml) vegetable broth or more 1 tablespoon (IS g) organic ketchup

2 teaspoons vegetable bouillon paste

1 tablespoon (15 ml) high heat neutral-flavored oil for cooking

For the cooking broth:

2 cups (470 ml) vegetable broth

1 tablespoon (IS g) organic ketchup 1 tablespoon (IS ml) tamari

1 teaspoon liquid smoke

¼ tsp pepper

1 tsp toasted sesame oil

Protein content per cutlet: 41 g

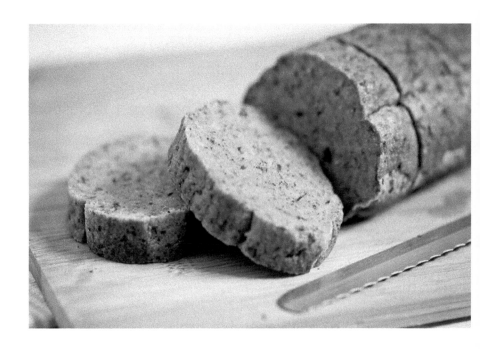

Harissa Seitan and Green Beans

Servings: 4

Ingredients:

1 tablespoon (15 ml) high heat neutral-flavored oil

8 ounces (227 g) Quit-the-Cluck Seitan, cut into ½-inch (1.3 cm) strips

2 handfuls green beans, trimmed, cut into bite-size pieces

½ of red pepper

1 leek, white part only, cut in half, sliced into half-rounds

½ cup (80 ml) dry red wine, or vegetable broth 1½ tablespoons (24 g) harissa paste, or to taste 3 tablespoons (48 g) tomato paste

1   cup (235 ml) vegetable broth

2   cloves garlic, minced Juice from ½ lemon Salt and pepper

Instructions:

1.   Put oil in a skillet. Bake for 5 minutes, occasionally stirring to brown.

2.   Cook beans for 3 minutes until they are green.

3.   Add the pepper and the leek and cook for 2 minutes, stirring to soften but not soft.

4.   Add a glass of wine (75 ml) of wine or broth to the pan and lower each bit. Reduce heat to medium.

5.   Add harissa paste, tomato paste, broth, garlic, and lemon juice. Stir to cover the olives and vegetables.

6.   Cook for 10 minutes, stirring occasionally. Season with salt and pepper.

Protein content per serving: 16 g

Easy Seitan for Two

Servings: 2

Ingredients:

½ teaspoon freshly ground black pepper Pinch of acceptable sea salt

2 (every 4 ounces, or 113 g) Kind-to- Cows Seitan cutlets 1/3 cup (80 ml) vegetable broth

1 tablespoon (16 g) tomato paste

1 teaspoon balsamic vinegar 1 teaspoon Dijon mustard

1 teaspoon white miso

1 tablespoon (15 ml) high heat neutral-flavored oil 2 tablespoons (20 g) minced shallot

Instructions

1.   Rub the pepper and salt evenly into the seitan cutlets.

2.   Whisk together the broth, tomato paste, vinegar, mustard, and miso in a small bowl.

3.   Heat the oil over medium-high heat in a large skillet.

4.   Put the cutlets into the skillet and cook for 3 to 5 minutes until browned. Turnover and cook the second side for 3 to 4 minutes until also browned. Remove the cutlets and set them aside.

5.   Reduce the heat to medium-low. Add the shallots. Cook and stir for 2 to 3 minutes, until softened. Be careful not to burn them. Scrap up any bits stuck to the skillet. Pour the broth mixture into the skillet. Bring to a simmer and stir for 3 to 4 minutes. Put the cutlets back into the skillet and turn to coat. Simmer for 3 and half minutes to heat the cutlets throughout. Spoon the sauce over the cutlets to serve.

Protein content per serving: 43 g

Pecan-Crusted Seitan Cutlets with Brussels Sprouts

Servings: 2

Ingredients

For the cutlets:

½ cup (120 ml) unsweetened plain vegan milk 3 tablespoons (42 g) vegan mayonnaise

1   tablespoon (15 g) Dijon mustard

¼ teaspoon acceptable sea salt, plus a pinch

½ teaspoon ground black pepper, plus a pinch

½ cup plus 2 tablespoons (63 g) pecan halves, ground 3 tablespoons (15 g) panko crumbs

¼ teaspoons onion powder

2   (every 4 ounces, or 113 g) Kind-to* Cows Seitan cutlets High heat neutral-flavored oil, for cooking

For the brussels sprouts:

1 tablespoon (15 ml) olive oil

12 ounces (340 g) of well- sliced Brussels sprouts 2 tablespoons (30 ml) vegetable broth

1 teaspoon Dijon mustard

3 tablespoons (21 g) grated carrots Salt and pepper

Instructions

1. To make the cutlets: Whisk together the milk, mayonnaise mustard, and a pinch each of salt and pepper in a shallow bowl. Combine the pecans, panko. Onion powder and remaining salt and pepper on a plate. Stir to combine. Line a baking sheet with parchment paper. Using one "wet" hand and one "dry" hand, dip each cutlet in the milk mixture, then in the pecan mixture, turning to coat thoroughly. Put on the lined baking sheet and repeat with the second cutlet. Refrigerate for 15 minutes or up to 8 hours. This helps to set the coating so it will not fall off during cooking.

2. To cook the cutlets, heat a thin layer of oil in a large, heavy-bottomed skillet. Cook the cutlets for 5 to 7 minutes until browned. Turnover and cook the second side for 4 to 6 minutes until also browned.

3.   To make the Brussels sprouts: Heat the oil in a large skillet over medium-high heat. Add the Brussels sprouts. Cook for 6 to 8 minutes, stirring occasionally. The Brussels sprouts should have some dark spots and be tender. Whisk broth and mustard in a small bowl. Turn the heat off. But leave the skillet on the weather. Stir in the broth mixture and the carrots. The liquid should evaporate or be absorbed — season to taste with salt and pepper.

4.   To serve, divide the Brussels sprouts between two plates and top, each with a cutlet.

Protein content per serving: 51 g

Sweet Potato and White Bean Skillet

Preparation Time: 5 minutes

 Cooking Time: 20 minutes

Servings: 4

Ingredients:

1   bunch kale, chopped

2   sweet potatoes, peeled, cubed 12 oz. cannellini beans

1 peeled onion, diced 1/8 tsp. Red pepper flakes 1 tsp. salt

1 tsp. Cumin

½ tsp. Ground black pepper 1 tsp. curry powder

1 ½ tbsps. coconut oil

6 oz. coconut milk, unsweetened

Directions:

1. Add ½ tablespoon oil on a skillet pan and when it melts, add onion and cook for 5 minutes.

2. Then stir in sweet potatoes, stir well, cook for 5 minutes, then season with all the spices, cook for 1 minute and remove the pan from heat.

3. Take another pan, add remaining oil in it, place it over medium heat and when oil melts, add kale, season with some salt and black pepper, stir well, pour in the milk, and cook for 15 minutes until tender.

4. Then add beans, beans, and red pepper, stir until mixed and cook for 5 minutes until hot.

5. Serve straight away.

Nutrition:

Calories: 263

Fat: 4 g

Carbs: 44 g Protein: 13g

Veggie Kabobs

Preparation Time: 10 minutes

Cooking Time: 10 minutes

Servings: 10

Ingredients:

8 oz. button mushrooms, halved

2 lbs. summer squash, peeled, 1-inch cubed 12 oz. small broccoli florets

2 cups grape tomatoes 1 tsp. Salt

½ tsp. Smoked paprika 1 tsp. ground cumin

6 tbsps. olive oil

1/2 tsp. ground coriander 1 lime, juiced

Directions:

1.   Toss broccoli florets with 1 tablespoon oil, toss tomatoes and squash pieces with 2 tablespoons oil, toss

mushrooms with 1 tablespoon oil and thread these vegetables onto skewers.

2.   Grill mushrooms and broccoli for 7 to 10 minutes, squash and tomatoes and 8 minutes, and when done, transfer the skewers to a plate and drizzle with lime juice and remaining oil.

3.   Prepared the spice mix, and for this, stir together salt, paprika, cumin, and coriander, sprinkle half of the mixture over grilled veggies, cover them with foil for 5 minutes, and then sprinkle with the remaining spice mix.

4.   Serve straight away.

Nutrition:

Calories: 112, Fat: 8g, Carbs: 7g, Protein: 4g

Pilaf with Garbanzos and Dried Apricots

Preparation Time: 5 minutes

Cooking Time: 20 minutes

Servings: 4

Ingredients:

1 cup bulgur

6 oz. cooked chickpeas

½ cup dried apricot

1 white onion, peeled, diced

½ tsps. Minced garlic 2 tsps. Curry powder

½ tsp. salt

1 tbsp. olive oil

¼ cup fresh parsley leaves 2 cups vegetable broth

¾ cup water

Directions:

1.	Take a saucepan, place it over high heat, pour in water and 1 ½ cup broth, and bring it to a boil.

2.	Then stir in bulgur, switch heat to medium-low level and simmer for 15 minutes until most of the liquid has absorbed.

3.	Meanwhile, take a skillet pan, place it over medium heat, add oil, and when hot, add onion, cook for 10 minutes, then stir in garlic and curry powder and cook for another minute.

4.	Then add apricots, beans, and salt, pour in the remaining broth, and bring the mixture to boiling.

5.	Remove pan from heat, fluff the bulgur with a fork, add to the onion-apricot mixture and stir until mixed.

6.	Garnish with parsley and serve.

Nutrition:

Calories: 222 Fat: 4.5g Carbs: 35g Protein: 9.5g

Spaghetti with Chickpeas Meatballs

Preparation Time: 10 minutes

Cooking Time: 40 minutes

Servings: 8

Ingredients:

½ cup Breadcrumbs

1 tsp. Italian Seasoning

3 cups Chickpeas, drained & rinsed

½ tsp. Salt

3 tbsps. Flax Seed grounded 2 tsps. Onion Powder

8 tbsps. Water

½ tbsp. Garlic Powder

¼ cup Nutritional Yeast For the pasta:

1 lb. Spaghetti

25 oz. Pasta Sauce

Directions:

1.   First, preheat the oven to 325°F.

2.   After that, combine the flax seeds with water in a small bowl and set them aside for 5 minutes.

3.   Next, place the chickpeas and salt in the food processor and process them for one minute or until you get a smooth mixture.

4.   Now, transfer the chickpea mixture and the flaxseed mixture to a large mixing bowl. Stir well.

5.   Once combined, add all the remaining ingredients needed to the bowl.

6.   Give everything a good stir and mix well.

7.   Then, make balls out of this mixture and arrange them on a parchment paper-lined baking sheet while leaving ample space in between.

8.   Bake them for 33 to 35 minutes. Turn them once halfway through.

9.   In the meantime, make the spaghetti by following the instructions given in the packet. Cook until al dente.

10.   Finally, place the spaghetti on the serving plate and top it with the meatballs and pasta sauce.

11.   Serve and enjoy.

Nutrition: Calories: 323, Proteins: 15g, Carbs: 63g, Fat: 4g

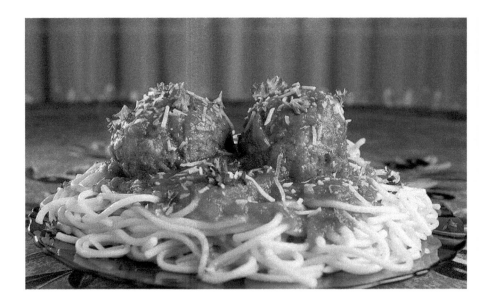

Black Bean Wrap with Hummus

Preparation Time: 5 minutes

Cooking Time: 30 minutes

Servings: 2 Wraps

Ingredients:

1   Poblano Pepper, roasted

½ packet Spinach 1 Onion, chopped

2   Whole Grain Wraps

½ can Black Beans

1 Bell Pepper, seeded & chopped

4 oz. Mushrooms, sliced

½ cup Corn

8 oz. Red Bell Pepper Hummus, roasted

Directions:

1.   First, preheat the oven to 450°F.

2.   Next, spoon in oil to a heated skillet and stir in the onion.

3.   Cook them for 2 to 3 minutes or until softened.

4.   After that, stir in the bell pepper and sauté for another 3 minutes.

5.   Then, add mushrooms and corn to the skillet. Sauté for 2 minutes.

6.   In the meantime, spread the hummus over the wraps.

7.   Now, place the sautéed vegetables, spinach, Poblano strips, and beans.

8.   Roll them into a burrito and place them on a baking sheet with the seam side down.

9.   Finally, bake them for 9 to 10 minutes.

10.   Serve them warm.

Nutrition:

Calories: 293, Proteins: 13.7g, Carbs: 42.8g, Fat: 8.8g

Sage Walnuts and Radishes

Preparation Time: 10 minutes

Cooking Time: 10 minutes

Servings: 6

Ingredients:

2   tablespoons olive oil 5 celery ribs, chopped

3   spring onions, chopped

½ pound radishes halved juice of 1 lime

Zest of 1 lime, grated

8 ounces walnuts, chopped A pinch of black pepper

3   tablespoons sage, chopped

Directions:

1. Add celery and spring onion to oil in a pan, stir and cook for 5 minutes.

2.   Add remainings ingredients, and cook for another 5 minutes, divide into bowls and serve.

Nutrition: calories 200 fat 7 fiber 5 carbs 9.3 protein 4

Grönsaksbullar (Swedish Vegan Meatballs)

Servings: 20 meatballs

Ingredients

For the meatballs:

115 g peas

1 and half onion

2 tbsp. rapeseed oil (plus extra for frying)

1 tsp ready-chopped garlic Protein content per serving garlic puree

2 and half carrots

1   red pepper

curly kale 400 g tin chickpeas

2   tbsp. olive oil

2 tbsp. nutritional yeast flakes (optional) 1 tsp vegetable stock powder

2 tbsp. gram flour

a little plain flour for dusting

For the sauce:

1 tbsp. Dairy-free margarine 1 tbsp. plain flour

200 ml dairy-free milk (soy, nut, or oat)

125 ml of boiling water

1 tsp vegetable stock powder

125 ml dairy-free cream (soy or oat) 2 tsp wholegrain mustard

soy sauce

Instructions

1.   Cook the peas in the microwave or a small pot for 2 minutes. Drain and set aside to cool.

2.   Peel the onion, cut it into quarters, and then use a mini crusher or a food chopper (or cut it by hand).

3.   Put oil on a large saucepan with oil and add the onions and garlic. Cook over medium heat.

4.   Peel the carrots and cut them into approximately 4-5 slices, then finely chop the crushed protein content in each food processor and add it to the onions. Then, chop the peppers in the same way, then cook the peas

and the curried cabbage. Let all the vegetables cook over medium heat.

5.   Drain and wash the chickpeas, then sprinkle with olive oil in a mini crusher or food processor in a nonstick skillet. Add to the pot, then sprinkle the yeast slices, the powdered broth, the warm flour, and a generous salt and pepper sauce. Mix all the ingredients, then remove from heat and let cool enough to cook.

6.   Sprinkle a handful of crushers and flour with a little flour, then glue a teaspoon of the mixture, wrap it tightly in a ball in your hand and place it on a crushing board. Repeat until the entire combination is used; It should have approximately 20 types of meat.

7.   Cover the bottom of a large pot with rapeseed or sunflower oil and fry the meatballs and turn until golden brown. Pour the cup into a plate covered with paper towels to drain the excess oil.

8.   Heat the margarine in a saucepan, stir the flour, and cook over medium heat for 2 minutes. Add non-dairy milk, water, powdered cream, and non-dairy cream and stir to mix until a thick and shiny sauce consistency is achieved. Add the mustard and stir. Add

drops of soy sauce and try everything you want so that the condiments do not reach the right level.

9.   Serve the meatballs with the sauce on top, with mashed potatoes or French fries.

Protein content per servings: 14.8 g

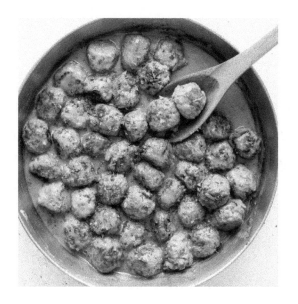

Chipotle Black Bean Chili with Nachos

Servings: 2

Ingredients

2 tbsp. rapeseed or sunflower oil 1 red onion

1 carrot

handful fresh coriander

1 tsp ready-chopped garlic Protein content per serving garlic puree 2-3 tsp chipotle paste (to your taste - 3 tsp is somewhat spicy)

1 red pepper

400 g tin black beans

400 g tin chopped tomatoes pinch sugar

salt and black pepper

Instructions

1.   Put a large bowl with oil. Peel the onions and carrots and remove the coriander stems from the leaves (remove them later).

2.   chop onions, carrots, and coriander. Use a mini crusher or food, and then add it to the pot.

3.   Add garlic and pea pasta to the pot and stir. Chop the seeds and finely chop the peppers and add them to the pan.

4.   Wash beans and add them to the pot.

5.   Chop the tomatoes and sugar, then season with salt and black pepper. Then cover it with a lid and heat it over high heat. Cook for 8-10 minutes, stirring constantly. Adjust and adjust seasoning if necessary.

6.   Chop the coriander leaves thoroughly and chop the peppers before serving with rice, fajita, or a handful of French fries.

7.   Heat the oil in a large pan. Half or a quarter of each giant mushroom, drop the smaller ones entirely and add them to the pot. Chop and chop the scallions and add to the pot with peanut nuts.

8.   Fill a pot with boiling water and add the noodles. Simmer for 5-6 minutes until freshly cooked. Drain and reserve.

9.   Mix the pepper sauce, soy sauce, and water with the smooth saucer.

10.   When the mushrooms are cooked and the peanuts are golden brown, pour the sauce into the pan and add the noodles when bubbling. Stir to combine, then serve immediately.

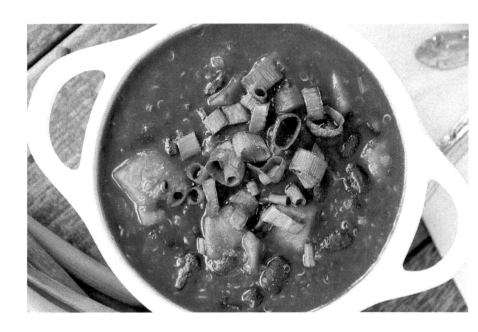

Exotic Mushroom & Cashew Sweet Chili Noodles

Servings: 2

Ingredients

2   tbsp. rapeseed or sunflower oil 200 g mixed 'exotic' mushrooms 4 spring onions

3   tbsp. cashew nuts

150 g (3 nests) whole-wheat noodles 3 tbsp. sweet chili sauce

2 tbsp. soy sauce

150 ml water

Instructions

1.   Make a large pan with oil. Peel the onions and carrots and remove the coriander stems from the leaves (remove them later). Chop onions, carrots, and coriander, use a mini crusher or food, and then add it to the pot.

2.   Add garlic and pea pasta to the pot and stir. Chop the seeds and finely chop the peppers and add them to the pan.

3.   Add beans to the pot. Chop the tomatoes and sugar, then season with salt and black pepper. Then cover it with a lid and heat it over high heat. Cook for 8-10

minutes,   stirring   constantly. Adjust   and adjust   seasoning   if necessary.

4.   Chop the coriander leaves thoroughly and chop the peppers before serving with rice, fajita, or a handful of French fries.

Koshari

Preparation Time: 15 minutes

Cooking Time: 2 hours 10 minutes

Servings: 6

Ingredients:

1 cup green lentils, rinsed 3 cups water

Salt, to taste (optional)

1   large onion, peeled and minced

2   tbsp vegetable broth

4 cloves garlic, peeled and minced

½ tsp allspice

1 tsp coriander

1 teaspoon ground cumin

2 tablespoons tomato paste

½ teaspoon crushed red pepper flakes 3 large tomatoes, diced

1 cup cooked medium-grain brown rice

1 cup whole-grain elbow macaroni, cooked, drained, and kept warm

1 tablespoon brown rice vinegar

Directions:

1.   Sprinkle lentils with salt, if desired. Bring to a boil over high heat. Reduce the heat to medium, then put the pan lid on and cook for 45 minutes or until the water is mostly absorbed. Pour the cooked lentils into the bowl and set them aside.

2.   Add the onion to a nonstick skillet, then sauté over medium heat for 15 minutes or caramelized.

3.   Add vegetable broth and garlic to the skillet and sauté for 3 minutes or until fragrant.

4.   Add the allspice, coriander, cumin, tomato paste, and red pepper flakes to the skillet and sauté for an additional 3 minutes until aromatic.

5.   Add the tomatoes to the skillet and sauté for 15 minutes or until the tomatoes are wilted. Sprinkle with salt, if desired.

6.   Arrange the cooked brown rice on the bottom of a large platter, then top the rice with macaroni, and then spread the lentils over. Pour the tomato mixture and brown rice vinegar over before serving.

Nutrition:

Calories: 201 Fat: 1.6g Carbs: 41.8g Protein: 6.5g Fiber: 3.6g

Black Bean & Sweet Potato Hash

Preparation Time: 5 minutes

Cooking Time: :20 minutes

Servings: 4 bowls

Ingredients:

1   cup onion

2 garlic cloves, minced

2   cups sweet potatoes, chopped and peeled 2 tsp hot chili powder

⅓ cup vegetable broth

1   cup cooked black beans

¼ cup chopped scallions Chopped cilantro, for Hot garnish sauce (optional)

Directions:

1.   In a nonstick skillet, place the onion and sauté over medium heat. Stir occasionally for 2 to 3 minutes. Add the garlic and stir.

2.   Add the chili pepper and sweet potatoes. Stir to coat the vegetables with chili powder.

3.   Add the broth and stir. Cook the contents for 12 minutes and occasionally stir until the potatoes are well-cooked.

4.   Add some liquid. This will keep the vegetables from sticking to the pan. Add the scallions, black beans, and salt. Cook for 1 and half minutes until the beans are well-heated.

5.   Add the hot sauce if you are using it. Stir. Check the taste and adjust accordingly with the seasoning.

6.   Top it with cilantro.

Nutrition:

Calories: 270 Fat: 7g Protein: 13g Carbs: 35g Fiber: 7g

Sweet and Salty Pineapple Fried Rice

Preparation Time: 5 minutes

Cooking Time: 15 minutes

Servings: 4

Ingredients:

Rice:

2   tbsp coconut oil

2/3 cup frozen green peas, thawed

½ cup sunflower seeds (raw) Red pepper (one large), diced

3   cups canned or fresh pineapple chunks 2 garlic cloves, minced

1   tbsp ginger, minced

2   cups long-grain brown rice, cooked Green onions (one bunch)

Sauce:

1 cup pineapple juice

4 tbsp tamari

1   tsp sesame oil

Lime juice (half a lime)

Chili sauce to taste (sriracha is a good option)

Directions:

1.   On medium heat in a large pan, toast the sunflower seeds for about 2 minutes. Set aside when the content is lightly browned.

2.   On medium heat using the same pan, heat the coconut oil. Add the red pepper, pineapple chunks, and 2/3 of the green onion. Stir for about 5 minutes.

3.   Now add the garlic and ginger. Stir so the tastes can meld.

4.   Keep the heat on high. Add the cold rice and cook for 5 minutes until it is toasty.

5.   Fold in the green peas as well as the toasted seeds

6.   With the pan still on medium heat, pour in the tamari, sesame oil, and pineapple juice. Stir.

7.   Season as required with the chili sauce.

8.   For a better taste, add more lime juice and salt as required.

Nutrition:

Calories: 180 Fat: 11g Protein: 18g Carbs: 38g Fiber: 12g

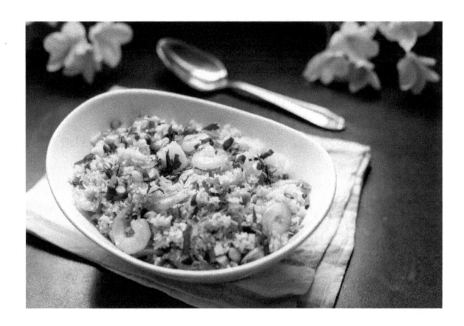

Black Bean Burgers

Preparation Time: 10 minutes

Cooking Time: 15 minutes

Servings: 6

Ingredients:

1   Onion, diced

½ cup Corn Nibs

2   Cloves Garlic, minced

½ teaspoon Oregano, dried

½ cup Flour

1   Jalapeno Pepper, small

2   cups Black Beans, mashed & canned

¼ cup Breadcrumbs (Vegan) 2 teaspoons Parsley, minced

¼ teaspoon cumin

1   tablespoon Olive Oil

2   teaspoons Chili Powder

½ Red Pepper, diced Sea Salt to taste

Directions:

1.   Set your flour on a plate, and then get out your garlic, onion, peppers, and oregano, throwing it in a pan. Cook over medium-high heat, and then cook until the onions are translucent. Place the peppers in, and sauté until tender.

2.   Cook for two minutes, and then set it to the side.

3.   Use a potato masher to mash your black beans, then stir in the vegetables, cumin, breadcrumbs, parsley, salt, and chili powder, and then divide it into six patties.

4.   Coat each side, and then cook until it is fried on each side.

Nutrition: Calories: 357 kcal Protein: 17.93 g Fat: 5.14 g Carbohydrates: 61.64 g

Dijon Maple Burgers

Preparation Time: 20 minutes

Cooking Time: 30 minutes

Servings: 12

Ingredients:

1 Red Bell Pepper

19 ounces Can be Chickpeas, rinsed & drained 1 cup Almonds, ground

2 teaspoons Dijon Mustard 1 teaspoon Oregano

½ teaspoon Sage

1 cup Spinach, fresh

1   – ½ cups Rolled Oats 1 Clove Garlic, pressed

½ Lemon, juiced

2   teaspoons Maple Syrup, pure

Directions: 1.   Get out a baking sheet. Line it with parchment paper.

2. Cut your red pepper in half, and then take the seeds out. Place it on your baking sheet and roast it in the oven while you prepare your other ingredients.

3. Process your chickpeas, almonds, mustard, and maple syrup together in a food processor.

4. Add in your lemon juice, oregano, sage, garlic, and spinach, processing again. Make sure it's combined, but don't puree it.

5. Once your red bell pepper is softened, which should roughly take ten minutes, add this to the processor as well. Add in your oats, mixing well.

6. Form twelve patties, cooking in the oven for a half-hour. They should be browned.

Nutrition: Calories: 96 kcal Protein: 5.28 g Fat: 2.42 g Carbohydrates: 16.82 g

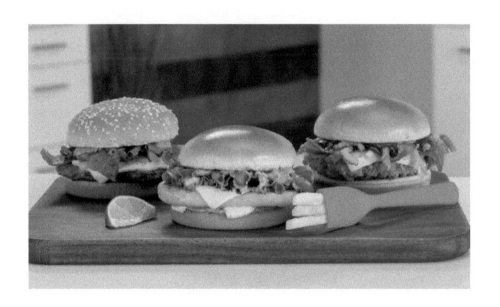

Hearty Black Lentil Curry

Preparation Time: 30 minutes

Cooking Time: 6 hours and 15 minutes

Servings: 4

Ingredients:

1   cup of black lentils, rinsed and soaked overnight
14 ounces of chopped tomatoes

2   large white onions, peeled and sliced 1 1/2
teaspoon of minced garlic

1 teaspoon of grated ginger 1 red chili

1 teaspoon of salt

1/4 teaspoon of red chili powder 1 teaspoon of paprika

1   tsp of turmeric

2 tsp of cumin

2   tsp of coriander

1/2 cup of chopped coriander

4-ounce of vegetarian butter 4 fluid of ounce water

2   fluid of ounce vegetarian double cream

Directions:

1.   Place a large pan over moderate heat, add butter and let heat until melt.

2.   Add the onion and garlic, and ginger and cook for 10 to 15 minutes or until onions are caramelized.

3.   Then stir in salt, red chili powder, paprika, turmeric, cumin, ground coriander, and water.

4.   Transfer this mixture to a 6-quart slow cooker and add tomatoes and red chili.

5.   Drain lentils, add to slow cooker, and stir until just mix.

6.   Plugin slow cooker; adjust cooking time to 6 hours and cook on low heat setting.

7.   When the   lentils   are   done, stir   in cream   and   adjust   the seasoning.

8.   Serve with boiled rice or whole wheat bread.

Nutrition: Calories: 299 kcal Protein: 5.59 g Fat: 27.92 g Carbohydrates: 9.83 g

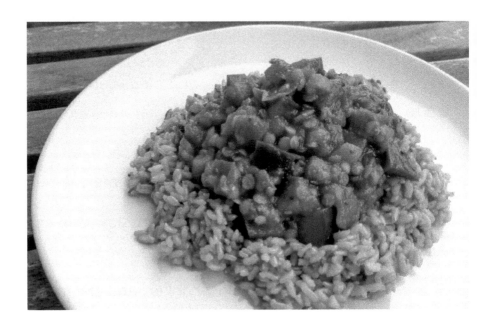

Flavorful Refried Beans

Preparation Time: 15 minutes

Cooking Time: 8 hours

Servings: 8

Ingredients:

3   cups of pinto beans, rinsed

1 jalapeno pepper

1 white onion,

2 tablespoons of minced garlic

5 teaspoons of salt

2 teaspoons of ground black pepper 1/4 teaspoon of ground cumin

9 cups of water

Directions: 1.   Using a 6-quart slow cooker, place all the ingredients and stir until it mixes properly.

2.   Cover the top, plug in the slow cooker, adjust the cooking time to 6 hours, let it cook on the high heat setting, and add more water if the beans get too dry.

3.   Drain the beans then reserve the liquid.

4.   Mash the beans and pour in the reserved cooking liquid until it reaches your desired mixture.

5.   Serve immediately.

Nutrition: Calories: 268 kcal Protein: 16.55 g Fat: 1.7 g Carbohydrates: 46.68 g

Smoky Red Beans and Rice

Preparation Time: 15 minutes

Cooking Time: 6 minutes

Servings: 6

Ingredients:

30 ounce of cooked red beans 1 cup of brown rice, uncooked 1 cup of chopped green pepper 1 cup of chopped celery

1 cup of chopped white onion 1 1/2 teaspoon of minced garlic 1/2 teaspoon of salt

1/4 teaspoon of cayenne pepper 1 teaspoon of smoked paprika 2 teaspoons of dried thyme

1   bay leaf

2   1/3 cups of vegetable broth

Directions: 1.   Using a 6-quart slow cooker, place all the ingredients except for the rice, salt, and cayenne pepper.

2.   Stir until it mixes appropriately, and then cover the top.

3.   Plug in the slow cooker, adjust the cooking time to 4 hours, and steam on a low heat setting.

4.   Then pour in and stir the rice, salt, cayenne pepper and continue cooking for an additional 2 hours at a high heat setting.

5.   Serve straight away.

Nutrition: Calories: 791 kcal Protein: 3.25 g Fat: 86.45 g Carbohydrates: 9.67 g

Comforting Chickpea Tagine

Preparation Time: 5 minutes

Cooking Time: 4 hours

Servings: 6

Ingredients:

14 oz. cooked chickpeas 12 dried apricots

1 red bell pepper, cored and sliced

1 cored butternut squash, peeled and chopped 2 stemmed zucchinis, chopped

1 white onion, peeled and chopped

1 tsp. Minced Garlic 1 tsp. Ground ginger 1 ½ tbsp. salt

1   tsp. Ground black pepper 1 tsp. ground cumin

2   tsps. paprika

1   tsp. Harissa paste 2 tsps. honey

2   tbsps. olive oil 1 lb. passata

¼ cup chopped coriander

Directions:

1.   Take a 6-quart slow cooker, grease it with a non-stick cooking spray and place the chickpeas, apricots, bell pepper, butternut squash, zucchini onion into it.

2.   Sprinkle it with salt, black pepper, and set it aside until it is called for.

3.   Place a large non-stick skillet pan over an average temperature of heat; add the oil, garlic, cumin, and paprika.

4.   Stir properly and cook for 1 minute or until it starts producing fragrance.

5.   Then pour in the harissa paste, honey, passata, and boil the mixture.

6.   When the mixture is done boiling, pour this mixture over the vegetables in the slow cooker and cover it with the lid.

7.   Plug in the slow cooker; adjust the cooking time to 4 hours and let it cook on the high heat setting or until the vegetables get tender.

8.   When done, add the seasoning, garnish it with the coriander, and serve right away.

Nutrition: Calories: 237 Carbs: 45g Protein: 9g Fat: 2g

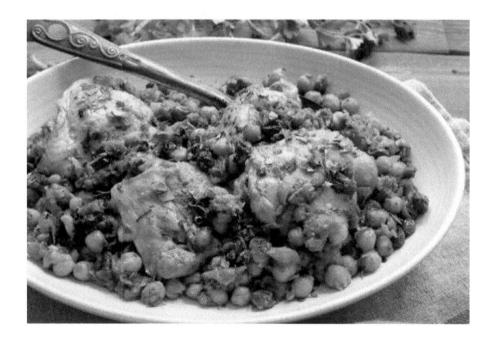

Black Bean Stuffed Sweet Potatoes

Preparation Time: 5 minutes

Cooking Time: 1 hour

Servings: 4

Ingredients:

4 sweet potatoes

15 oz. Cooked black beans

½ tsp. Ground black pepper

½ red onion, peeled, diced

½ tsp. Sea salt

¼ tsp. Onion powder

¼ tsp. Garlic powder

¼ tsp. Red chili powder

¼ tsp. cumin

1 tsp. lime juice

1 ½ tbsps. olive oil

½ cup cashew cream sauce

Directions:

1. Spread sweet potatoes on a baking tray greased with foil and bake for 65 minutes at 350°F until tender.

2. Meanwhile, prepare the sauce, and for this, whisk together the cream sauce, black pepper, and lime juice until combined, set aside until required.

3. When 10 minutes of the baking time of potatoes are left, heat a skillet pan with oil. Add in the onion to cook until golden for 5 minutes.

4. Then stir in spice, cook for another 3 minutes, stir in bean until combined, and cook for 5 minutes until hot.

5. Let roasted sweet potatoes cool for 10 minutes, then cut them open, mash the flesh, and top with bean mixture, cilantro, and avocado, and then drizzle with cream sauce.

Nutrition: Calories: 387, Fat: 16.1 g, Carbs: 53 g, Protein: 10.4g

Black Bean and Quinoa Salad

Preparation Time: 10 minutes

Cooking Time: 0 minute

Servings: 10

Ingredients:

15 oz. cooked black beans

1 chopped red bell pepper, cored 1 cup quinoa, cooked

1   cored green bell pepper, chopped

½ cup vegan feta cheese, crumbled

Directions:

1.   In a bowl, set in all ingredients, except for cheese, and stir until incorporated.

2.   Top the salad with cheese and serve straight away.

Nutrition: Calories: 64, Fat: 1g, Carbs: 8g, Protein: 3g

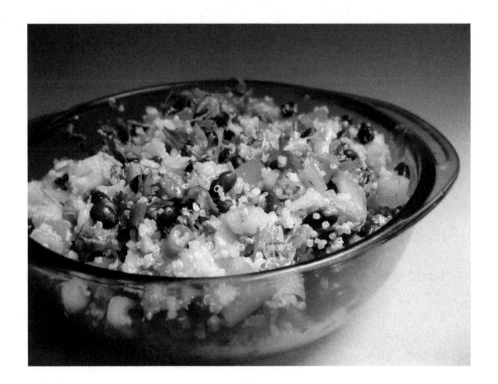

Coconut Chickpea Curry

Preparation Time: 5 minutes

Cooking Time: 15 minutes

Servings: 4

Ingredients:

2   tsps. coconut flour

16 oz. Cooked chickpeas 14 oz. tomatoes, diced

1 red onion, sliced

1 ½ tsps. Minced garlic

½ tsp. sea salt

1 tsp. curry powder

1/3 tsp. Ground black pepper 1 ½ tbsps. garam masala

¼ tsp. cumin 1 lime, juiced

13.5 oz. Coconut milk, unsweetened 2 tbsps. coconut oil

Directions:

1.   Add oil to a large pot and when it melts, add onions and tomatoes, season with salt and black pepper, and cook for 5 minutes.

2.   Switch heat to medium-low level, cook for 10 minutes until tomatoes have released their liquid, then add chickpeas and stir in garlic, curry powder, garam masala, and cumin until combined.

3.   Stir in milk and flour, bring the mixture to boil, switch heat to medium heat and simmer the curry for 12 minutes until cooked.

4.   Taste to adjust seasoning, drizzle with lime juice, and serve.

Nutrition:

Calories: 225

Fat: 9.4 g Carbs: 28.5g Protein: 7.3g

Garlic Zucchini and Cauliflower

Preparation Time: 10 minutes

Cooking Time: 20 minutes

Servings: 4

Ingredients:

4   zucchinis, cut into medium fries 1 cup cauliflower florets

1 tablespoon capers, drained Juice of ½ lemon

A pinch of salt and black pepper

½ teaspoon chili powder 1 tablespoon olive oil

¼ teaspoon garlic powder

Directions:

1.   Spread the zucchini fries on a lined baking sheet, add the rest of the ingredients, toss, introduce in the oven, bake at 400 degrees F for 20 minutes, divide between plates and serve.

Nutrition: calories 185 fat 3 fiber 2 carbs 6.5 protein 8

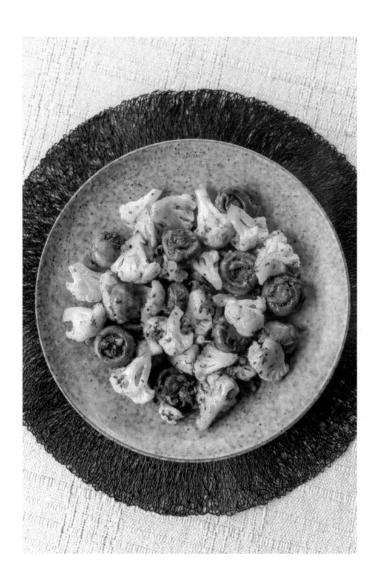

Garlic Beans

Preparation Time: 10 minutes

Cooking Time: 10 minutes

Servings: 4

Ingredients:

Juice of 1 lemon

Zest of 1 lemon, grated

2 tbsp avocado oil

4 garlic cloves

½ teaspoon turmeric powder 1 teaspoon garam masala

1 red onion, sliced

1 yellow bell pepper, sliced 10 ounces green beans, halved

A pinch of black pepper

Directions:

1.   Add the garlic and onion to oil and cook for 2 minutes.

2.   Add green beans and the other ingredients, toss, cook for 8 minutes, divide between plates and serve.

Nutrition: calories 180 fat 10 fiber 6 carbs 13 protein 8

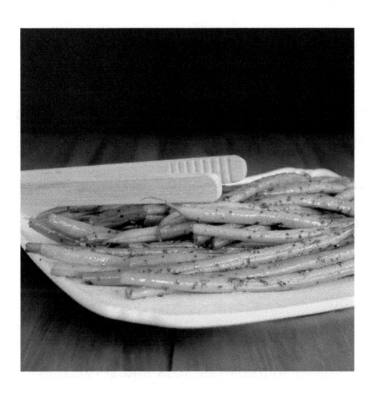

Mustard Beets

Preparation Time: 10 minutes

Cooking Time: 0 minutes

Servings: 4

Ingredients:

1 tablespoon Dijon mustard 1 and ½ tablespoon olive oil

8 ounces beets, cooked and sliced 1 teaspoon garam masala

1 teaspoon coriander, ground 1 teaspoon basil, dried

A pinch of black pepper

Directions:

1.   In a bowl, mix the beets with the oil, mustard, and the other ingredients, toss and serve.

Nutrition: calories 170 fat 5 fiber 7 carbs 8 proteins 5.5

Parsley Green Beans

Preparation Time: 10 minutes

Cooking Time: 20 minutes

Servings: 6

Ingredients:

3 tablespoons olive oil

3 pounds green beans, halved

Salt and black pepper

2 tbps balsamic vinegar 2 yellow onions, chopped

2 and ½ tablespoons parsley, chopped

Directions:

1.   Add the green beans and the other ingredients to oil, toss, cook for 20 minutes, divide between plates and serve.

Nutrition: calories 130 fat 1 fiber 2 carbs 7.4 protein 6

Squash and Tomatoes

Preparation Time: 15 minutes

Cooking Time: 12 minutes

Servings: 2

Ingredients:

8 oz yellow squash, peeled and roughly cubed 1 cup cherry tomatoes, halved

3 tablespoons tomato sauce 1 teaspoon sweet paprika

1 teaspoon coriander, ground 1 teaspoon oregano, dried

1 teaspoon olive oil

1 teaspoon white pepper

Directions:

1.   Add the squash, tomatoes, and the other ingredients to oil, toss, cook for 12 minutes, divide between plates and serve.

Spicy Black-Eyed Peas

Preparation Time: 12 minutes

Cooking Time: 8 hours and 8 minutes

Servings: 8

Ingredients:

32-ounce black-eyed peas, uncooked 1 cup of chopped orange bell pepper 1 cup of chopped celery

8-ounce of chipotle peppers, chopped 1 cup of chopped carrot

1 cup of chopped white onion 1 teaspoon of minced garlic 3/4 teaspoon of salt

1/2 teaspoon of ground black pepper 2 teaspoons of liquid smoke flavoring 2 teaspoons of ground cumin

1 tablespoon of adobo sauce 2 tablespoons of olive oil

1 tablespoon of apple cider vinegar 4 cups of vegetable broth

Directions:

1.   Place a medium-sized non-stick skillet pan over an average temperature of heat; add the bell peppers, carrot, onion, garlic, oil, and vinegar.

2.   Stir until it mixes properly and let it cook for 5 to 8 minutes or until it gets translucent.

3.   Transfer this mixture to a 6-quarts slow cooker and add the peas, chipotle pepper, adobo sauce, and vegetable broth.

4.   Stir until appropriately mixed and cover the top.

5.   Plug in the slow cooker, adjust the cooking time to 8 hours, and let it cook on the low heat setting or until peas are soft.

6.   Serve right away.

Nutrition: Calories: 1071 kcal Protein: 5.3 g Fat: 113.65 g Carbohydrates: 18.51 g

Creamy Artichoke Soup

Preparation Time: 5 minutes

Cooking Time: 40 minutes

Servings: 4

Ingredients:

1   can artichoke hearts, drained 3 cups vegetable broth

2   tbsp. lemon juice

1   small onion, finely cut 2 cloves garlic, crushed 3 tbsp. olive oil

2   tbsp. flour

½ cup vegan cream

Directions:

1.   Gently sauté the onion and garlic in some olive oil. Add the flour, whisking constantly, and then add the

hot vegetable broth slowly while still whisking. Cook for about 5 minutes.

2.   Blend the artichoke, lemon juice, salt, and pepper until smooth. Add the puree to the broth mix, stir well, and then stir in the cream. Cook until heated through. Garnish with a swirl of vegan cream or a sliver of artichoke.

Nutrition: Calories: 1622 kcal Protein: 4.45 g Fat: 181.08 g Carbohydrates: 10.99 g

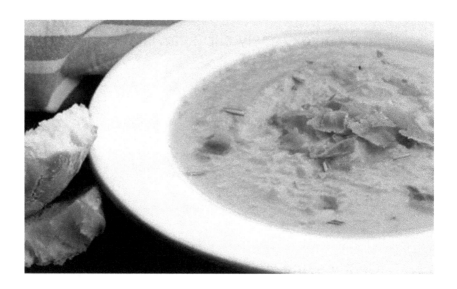

Tomato Artichoke Soup

Preparation Time: 5 minutes

Cooking Time: 35 minutes

Servings: 4

Ingredients:

1 can artichoke hearts

1 can diced tomatoes

3 cups vegetable broth

2 cloves garlic, crushed 1 tbsp. pesto

Black pepper, to taste

1 small onion, chopped

Directions:

1.   Combine all ingredients in the slow cooker.

2. Cook on low for 9 hours or on high for 4-5 hours.

3.   Blend the soup in batches, then put it back in the slow cooker. Season with pepper and salt, then serve.

Nutrition: Calories: 1487 kcal Protein: 3.98 g Fat: 167.42 g Carbohydrates: 8.2 g

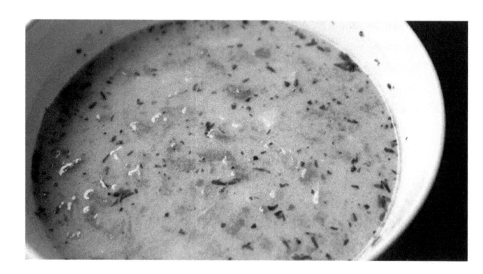

Super Radish Avocado Salad

Preparation Time: 10 minutes

Cooking Time: 25 minutes

Servings: 2

Ingredients:

6 shredded carrots

6 ounces diced radishes 1 diced avocado

1/3 cup ponzu

Directions:

1.   Place all together with the ingredients in a serving bowl and toss. Enjoy!

Nutrition: Calories: 292 kcal Protein: 7.42 g Fat: 18.29 g Carbohydrates: 29.59 g

Quit-the-Cluck Seitan

Servings: 6 (4 ounces, or 113 g each)

For the seitan:

1¼ cups (150 g) vital wheat gluten

¼ cup (30 g) chickpea flour

3 tablespoons (22 g) nutritional yeast

1   tablespoon (7 g) onion powder

2   teaspoons dried poultry seasoning

1   teaspoon garlic powder

½ teaspoon ground white pepper

¼ cup (180 ml) vegetable broth

2   teaspoons no chicken bouillon paste 1 tablespoon (15 ml) olive oil

1   tablespoon high heat neutral-flavored oil for cooking

For the cooking broth:

2   cups (470 ml) vegetable broth

1 tablespoon (8 g) nutritional yeast 2 teaspoons dried poultry seasoning 2 teaspoons onion powder

1 teaspoon Dijon mustard Salt and pepper

Instructions

To make the seitan:

1.   Put the oven to 320°F

2.   Stir the dry ingredients together in a medium-sized bowl. Stir the wet ingredients together in a measuring cup.

3.   Pour the wet ingredients into the dry ingredients and stir to combine. Knead with your hands until it forms a cohesive ball.

4.   Add tablespoon vital wheat gluten (9 g) or broth (15 ml), if needed, to reach the desired consistency. Divide into 6 equal portions.

5.   Sandwich a portion of dough between two pieces of parchment paper.

6.   Roll each portion into a cutlet that is no more than 1/2 inch (1.3 cm) thick.

7.   Put oil on a skillet. Cook the cutlets for 3 and half minutes until browned.

8.   Turnover and cook the second side for 3 minutes until browned.

 To prepare the cooking broth:

9.   Stir all the ingredients together in a 9 x 13 inch (22 x 23 cm) baking dish.

10.   Put the cutlets in the broth and cover the pan tightly with foil. Bake for 1 hour.

11.   Turn off the oven and let the seitan sit in the oven for 1 hour.

12.   Cool the seitan in the broth. Store the seitan and the broth for up to 3 days or freeze for up to two months.

Protein content per cutlet: 41 g

Best Baked Tofu and Kale

Servings: 4

Ingredients:

¼ cup wheat pastry flour or all-purpose flour

½ teaspoon ground white pepper

1   recipe Best Baked Tofu prepared

2   tablespoons (30 ml) high heat neutral-flavored oil

3 cloves garlic, thinly sliced

¼ cup (40 g) minced shallot

2 tablespoons (7 g) minced sun-dried tomatoes 4 cups (268 g) kale, chopped

1   can diced tomatoes

½ cup (120 ml) vegetable broth

½ cup (60 ml) dry white wine

2   tablespoons (5 g) chopped fresh basil Juice from ½ lemon

Salt and pepper

Instructions

1.   Preheat the oven to 350°F (180°C. or gas mark 4). Combine the flour and pepper on a plate. Coat the baked tofu slices with the mixture.

2.   Heat the oil in a large skillet over medium-high heat.

3.   Cook the tofu slices (in batches) for 3 to 4 minutes until browned. Turn over to cook the second side for 3 to 4 minutes until also browned. Put the tofu in the oven to keep warm.

4.   In the same skillet, cook the garlic, shallot, and a pinch of salt over medium heat for 3 to 4 minutes, until fragrant. Add the sun-dried tomatoes, kale, tomatoes, broth, and wine (if using). Bring to a simmer, and then cook for 12 to 15 minutes until the kale is tender. Stir in the basil and lemon juice and season to taste with salt and pepper. Serve the tofu slices on top of the greens.

Protein content per serving: 19 g

Broccoli & Walnut Pesto

Servings: 4

Ingredients

For the pesto:

1   head broccoli, cut into florets 75 g walnut pieces

2   cloves garlic

juice of 1 lemon 2 tbsp. olive oil

For the Pasta Alia Genovese:

500 g pasta

1 large floury potato, peeled and sliced fairly thinly

200 g fine green beans

Instructions

1.   Boil a large pot of water, then add the broccoli
and cook for 5-6 minutes. Remove with a slotted spoon
and place in the blender.

2.   Add the pasta and potato slices to the pot and boil again. Cook for 8 minutes, then add the green beans and cook for another 2 minutes or until the pasta is cooked.

3.   (Potato slices break while cooking, don't panic, imagine!).

4.   Meanwhile, add nuts, garlic, lemon, and olive oil to the mixture with broccoli and cabbage to mix. Season generously with salt and pepper, add a little water, cut again, and continue cooking until it reaches a consistency similar to the sauce.

5.   Drain the pasta, potatoes, and beans, then return to the pot and stir through the broccoli plague. Heat the oven over low heat and stir to remove the pest.

6.   Serve immediately!

Broccoli, Kale, Chili & Hazelnut Pizza

Servings: 2 large pizzas

Ingredients

500 g Whole Meal Bread Mix 200 ml Passata with Garlic

1 red onion, peeled and finely sliced

6 sun-dried tomatoes, roughly chopped

75 g fresh curly kale, woody stalks removed, and leaves roughly chopped

6-8 stalks purple sprouting broccoli, the lower half of stalks removed

1 red chili, finely sliced

handful hazelnuts, roughly chopped dried oregano

black pepper

extra virgin olive oil

Instructions

1.   Pack the bread mix according to the instructions. Kneel and let it grow in a warm place for 45.45 minutes.

2.   Meanwhile, prepare the meatballs and heat the oven to 200 degrees Celsius at 400 degrees C with protein content per serving of 6 gasoline and put it in the oven if using a pizza stone. (Check if your stove has a specific pizza setting, many do, which makes a big difference).

3.   Spread the dough on a floured surface and divide it in two. Insert each section into a ground ball and then roll with a roller in a 30 cm circle.

4.   When all the tanks are ready, and the stove is at maximum temperature, remove the pizza from the oven (or grease a baking sheet) or place the dough on the stone surface. Protein on each plate, cover with half the pasta, then the onion. Sprinkle with cabbage, broccoli, peppers, and hazelnuts, then sprinkle with mint and black pepper and sprinkle with olive oil. Repeat for the second pizza.

5.   Bake for 8-10 minutes until the slices brown and the base is well cooked.

Rice & Veggie Bowl

Preparation Time: 5 minutes

Cooking Time: 15 minutes

Servings: 6

Ingredients:

2   tbsp coconut oil 1 tsp ground cumin

1 tsp ground turmeric 1 tsp chili powder

1 red bell pepper, chopped 1 tsp tomato paste

1 bunch of broccoli, with short stems 1 tsp salt, to taste

1 onion

2 garlic cloves, minced

1 head of cauliflower, cut into bite-sized florets 2 cups cooked rice (or other cooked grain) Freshly ground black pepper to taste

Directions:

1.   In a large pan or skillet, heat the coconut oil over medium-high heat.

2.   When the oil is hot, stir in the turmeric, cumin, chili powder, salt, and tomato paste.

3.   Cook the content for 1 minute. Stir repeatedly until the spices are fragrant.

4.   Add the garlic and onion. Sauté for 2 and half minutes until the onions are softened.

5.   Add the broccoli, cauliflower, and bell pepper. Cover. Cook for 3 to 4 minutes and stir occasionally.

6.   Add the cooked rice. Stir so it will combine well with the vegetables. Cook for 2 to 3 minutes. Stir until the rice is warmed through.

7.   Adjust to taste

8.   Lower the heat and cook on low for 2 to 3 more minutes so the flavors will meld.

9.   Serve with freshly ground black pepper.

Nutrition:

Calories: 260 Fat: 9g Protein: 9g Carbs: 36g Fiber: 5g

Red Beans and Rice

Preparation Time: 5 minutes

Cooking Time: 25 minutes

Servings: 4

Ingredients:

3½ cups water, divided 1 tsp red pepper flakes 3 stalks celery, diced

1   green pepper, chopped

½ yellow onion, diced

2   small cans of kidney beans, drained and rinsed 1 cup brown rice

3   garlic cloves, minced 1 bay leaf

1 tsp sage

½ tsp oregano

½ tsp cayenne

Optional for heat: 1-2 jalapenos, diced

Directions:

1.   Add 1 cup of rice and 2 cups of water to a pot. Bring the contents to a boil, cover to simmer until the water is absorbed.

2.   Once the rice is cooked, put all the remaining ingredients in a large saucepan and cover 20 to 30 minutes on low-medium heat. Stir occasionally until the onions are cooked, and the 1 cup of water has boiled off.

Nutrition:

Calories: 221 Fat: 1g Protein: 11g Carbs: 25g Fiber: 4g

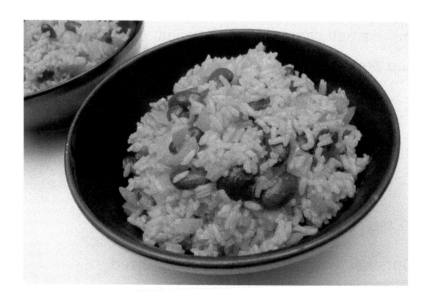

Raw Noodles with Avocado 'N Nuts

Preparation Time: 5 minutes

Cooking Time: 10 minutes

Servings: 2

Ingredients:

1 zucchini 1½ cup basil 1/3 cup water

5 tbsps. pine nuts

2 tbsps. lemon juice

1 avocado, peeled, pitted, sliced Optional: 2 tbsps. olive oil

6 yellow cherry tomatoes, halved Optional: 6 red cherry tomatoes, halved Sea salt, and black pepper

Directions:

1.   Add the basil, water, nuts, lemon juice, avocado slices, optional olive oil (if desired), salt, and pepper to a blender.

2.   Blend the ingredients into a smooth mixture. Season with more pepper and salt and blend again.

3.   Divide the sauce and the zucchini noodles between two medium-sized bowls for serving, and combine in each.

4.   Top the mixtures with the halved yellow cherry tomatoes and the optional red cherry tomatoes (if desired);

Nutrition:

Calories: 317, Carbs: 7.4 g, Fat: 28.1 g, Protein: 7.2g

Rice & Bean Burritos

Preparation Time: 10 minutes

Cooking Time: 15 minutes

Servings: 8

Ingredients:

32 oz. fat-free refried beans 6 tortillas

2 cups cooked rice

½ cup salsa

1 tbsp. olive oil

1 bunch green onions, chopped 2 bell peppers, chopped
Guacamole

Directions:

1.   Preheat the oven to 375°F.

2.   Dump the refried beans into a saucepan and place over medium heat to warm.

3.   Heat the tortillas and lay them out on a flat surface.

4.   Spoon the beans in a long mound that runs across the tortilla, just a little off from the center.

5.   Spoon some rice and salsa over the beans; add the green pepper and onions to taste, along with any other finely chopped vegetables you like.

6.   Fold over the shortest edge of the plain tortilla and roll it up, folding in the sides as you go.

7.   Place each burrito, seam side down, on a nonstick-sprayed baking sheet.

8.   Brush with olive oil and bake for 15 minutes.

Nutrition:

Calories: 290, Carbs: 49 g, Fat: 6 g, Protein: 9g

Lightning Source UK Ltd.
Milton Keynes UK
UKHW022008030521
383075UK00003B/326

9 781802 692198